Disclaimer

This book is intended to help people become consumers. The information in this book is intended to suppｏ not replace, the medical advice of a trained health care professional. No mention or description of uses of drugs listed herein should be construed as an endorsement of those uses or drugs. Only a physician can prescribe drugs and their precise dosages. All matters regarding your health require medical supervision. The authors and publisher disclaim any liability arising directly or indirectly from use of this book.

Notice of rights

Trademarks

Table of Contents

Your feedback is invaluable to us

If you recently bought this book, we would love to hear from you! You can do this by writing a review on amazon (or the online store where you purchased this book) about your last purchase! As part of our continual service improvement process, we love to hear real client experiences and feedback.

How does it work?
To post a review on Amazon, just log in to your account and click on the Create Your Own Review button (under Customer Reviews) of the relevant product page. You can find examples of product reviews in Amazon. If you purchased from another online store, simply follow their procedures.

Why use this book?

Everyone should ask questions when getting a prescription. This is especially important when your doctor or other health care professional prescribes you Terbinafine (OTC).

What should you ask?

Your health depends on good communication, but which questions to ask your doctor? Having the right questions is the answer.

Asking questions and providing information to your doctor and other care providers can improve your care. Talking with your doctor builds trust and leads to better satisfaction, quality, safety and results.

Asking questions is key to good communication with your doctor. If you do not ask questions, he or she may assume you already know the answer or that you do not want more information. Do not wait for the doctor to raise a specific question or subject; he or she may not know it is important to you. Be proactive. Ask questions.

Effective health care is a team effort. You are part of this team and play an important role. One of the best ways to communicate with your doctor and health care team is by asking questions. Since time is limited when you have your medical appointments, you will feel less rushed when you prepare your questions before your appointment.

Your doctor wants your questions. Doctors know a lot about a lot of things, but they do not always know everything about you, what you want to know or what is best for you.

Your questions give your doctor and health care professionals important information about you, like your most important health care concerns.

That is why they need you to speak up.

How to use this book?

When you meet with your doctor or other members of your health care team, you will hear a lot of information. It helps to think ahead of time of the things you want to know and to highlight the questions in this book you want to ask and take this book with you to your appointments.

This book contains questions you may want to ask your doctor. You should use the questions that fit your situation, and skip those that do not apply.

This book offers many ways that you can ask questions and get your health care needs met. With this book you will have numerous simple questions that can help you take better care of yourself, feel better, and get the right care at the right time.

Doctors and medical professionals want to know your questions to help them take better care of you and offer advice to get your most pressing questions answered.

Be prepared for your next medical appointment. Take this book with you if you are getting a checkup, want to discuss a problem or health condition, are getting a prescription, or talk about a medical test or surgery and be sure to write down the answers your health care professional provides for you in this book.

Whatever the reason for your appointment, it is important to be prepared.

Take charge of your health. Ask your health care providers questions and learn about the Terbinafine (OTC) medicine you take.

BEGINNING OF THE
QUESTION CHAPTERS:

CHAPTER #1: WHO:

INTENT: Who benefits from Terbinafine
(OTC) (Is this right for me.)

1. Who is validating my Terbinafine (OTC) prescription drugs to make sure I am taking the correct pills?

Notes:

2. Are there any side effects from taking nutritional supplements and Terbinafine (OTC) prescription medications at the same time?

Notes:

3. Is this worth getting Terbinafine (OTC) medication for?

Notes:

4. Is there anything I should do to help prevent my health issue?

Notes:

5. May my employer ask me which Terbinafine (OTC) prescription medications I am taking?

Notes:

6. Who is qualified to receive Terbinafine (OTC) prescription drug help?

Notes:

7. Who typically uses Terbinafine (OTC) prescription drugs, and where do they get them?

Notes:

8. How do you prevent re-admission in case I forget to take my Terbinafine (OTC) prescription medications. How do you help those who have problems following suggestions regarding eating habits, smoking, drinking, and taking drugs..?

Notes:

9. Are there safe Terbinafine (OTC)-class prescription drugs available?

Notes:

10. Is there financial help for Terbinafine (OTC) prescription drugs?

Notes:

11. Have you heard any stories about buying Terbinafine (OTC) prescription drugs over the internet?

Notes:

12. When in care who is responsible for the MAR (Medication Administration Records), who can put information on to it and make changes?

Notes:

13. Should I bring my Terbinafine (OTC) medications with me everywhere I go?

Notes:

14. Can I take Terbinafine (OTC) with prescription medication or with an underlying medical condition?

Notes:

15. If the pharmacist offers me a different brand of the same Terbinafine (OTC)-like medicine - is it ok to take it?

Notes:

16. Who can join a Medicare Terbinafine (OTC) prescription drug plan?

Notes:

17. If I am unable to comply with the treatment regimen, who else can administer Terbinafine (OTC) medication?

Notes:

18. What if I refuse the prescribed Terbinafine (OTC) medication?

Notes:

19. Has there been any follow up of those who have stopped taking Terbinafine (OTC) medication?

Notes:

20. Will Terbinafine (OTC) prescriptions drugs affect urine drug screen?

Notes:

21. If I get concerned with the high cost of medical care and Terbinafine (OTC) prescriptions drugs, will you help me explore my options for a more natural approach like seeking help from acupuncturists, naturopaths, chiropractors?

Notes:

22. What is the safest prescription drug disposal method?

Notes:

23. I am paid to _____ for a living, will my

performance improve or decrease while using Terbinafine (OTC) prescription drugs?

Notes:

24. Can a Terbinafine (OTC) prescription drug card preserve me cash?

Notes:

25. Will I have to take my medications forever?

Notes:

26. What if I start depending on antidepressants, alcohol, or other medications to calm me down or help me sleep?

Notes:

27. Do I need medication or surgery?

Notes:

28. Are extended-release (ER) opioid medications optimum pain medications?

Notes:

29. Do individual policies pay for prescription Terbinafine (OTC) medications?

Notes:

30. Which medication for my condition is right for me?

Notes:

31. What is your opinion on Terbinafine (OTC) prescription medications , side effects and IBS?

Notes:

32. Does my plan cover the Terbinafine (OTC) prescription drugs I need?

Notes:

33. Do you know of any natural medication to help?

Notes:

34. Which Terbinafine (OTC)-related prescription drugs are most dangerous?

Notes:

35. Who is at risk for Terbinafine (OTC) prescription drug addiction?

Notes:

36. I am feeling anxious and/or blue lately. Is this normal, can you help me?

Notes:

37. What if my religion condones the use of Terbinafine (OTC) medications?

Notes:

38. Are there any co-pays for medical treatments, hospitalization or Terbinafine (OTC) prescription drugs?

Notes:

39. Has anyone ever used this Terbinafine (OTC) medication?

Notes:

40. So who approves these Terbinafine (OTC) medications?

Notes:

41. Are side effects from Terbinafine (OTC) medications the same in males and females?

Notes:

42. How do you help someone who has a Terbinafine (OTC) prescription drugs addiction?

Notes:

43. Who is accountable for my Terbinafine (OTC) prescription drug use?

Notes:

44. Who can assist with Terbinafine (OTC) medication reminders?

Notes:

45. Do I really need this test?

Notes:

46. What are the Terbinafine (OTC) prescription drug prices?

Notes:

47. Are herbal supplements safe when I am taking other Terbinafine (OTC) prescription medications?

Notes:

48. Who gets to see the Terbinafine (OTC) prescription drug information submitted in my patient medical questionnaire?

Notes:

49. Who makes this Terbinafine (OTC) medication?

Notes:

50. Are there any other medicines that can help me but without any side effects?

Notes:

51. What can I expect about the absorption of active ingredients in my Terbinafine (OTC) prescription medications?

Notes:

52. Will I need any Terbinafine (OTC) medication after surgery?

Notes:

53. Who is eligible to receive Terbinafine (OTC) prescription drug help?

Notes:

54. Is Terbinafine (OTC) a medication?

Notes:

55. Can natural be just as potent, if not more potent than over-the-counter drugs, creams and ointments?

Notes:

56. What are the effects of Terbinafine (OTC) medications on cognition?

Notes:

57. Who can get Medicare Terbinafine (OTC) prescription drug coverage?

Notes:

58. Are related potential conditions avoidable, or do they require topical or other prescription medications?

Notes:

59. What if I am affected by anxiety and don't like the thought of taking prescription medications?

Notes:

60. What are the differences between generic and brand medications?

Notes:

61. Is there any form of exercise or medication you can recommend to enhance the effects of Terbinafine (OTC)?

Notes:

62. Who gets Terbinafine (OTC), and when?

Notes:

63. Which Terbinafine (OTC) prescription drugs can be addictive?

Notes:

64. Do I have to pay for my own Terbinafine (OTC) prescription drugs?

Notes:

65. Is this normal or should I see a shrink for Terbinafine (OTC) medication?

Notes:

66. Can and should I continue my Terbinafine (OTC) medication while on a weight loss diet?

Notes:

67. Who can I contact if I want to meet with a specialist for long-term Terbinafine (OTC) medication management on an ongoing basis?

Notes:

68. Who should NOT take Terbinafine (OTC) medication?

Notes:

69. Are my prescription drugs also available in a generic version?

Notes:

70. Is there anything else I should be asking?

Notes:

71. What is the difference between a natural herbal supplement and a prescription drug?

Notes:

72. Are there any risks involved in having this test?

Notes:

73. Will Terbinafine (OTC) cause me to test positive for various substances in a urine drug test?

Notes:

74. Can I share Terbinafine (OTC) prescription drugs?

Notes:

75. Who typically, signed up for the Medicare Prescription Drug plan, are already hitting the gap in coverage known as the doughnut hole - and what is my risk of hitting the doughnut hole?

Notes:

76. How can I get Terbinafine (OTC) prescription drug coverage?

Notes:

77. Are there any side effects of taking Terbinafine (OTC)?

Notes:

78. How can a wholesome mud-bath help my condition, and what is the effect on my Terbinafine (OTC) prescription drugs?

Notes:

79. Is it likely to get worse, or is it likely to get better?

Notes:

80. Who is most susceptible to Terbinafine (OTC) prescription drug abuse?

Notes:

81. They say _____ not to take this with Terbinafine (OTC) prescription medication, but do you think it will hurt me?

Notes:

82. Where I can get a Terbinafine (OTC) prescription drug?

Notes:

83. What is the Prescription Drug Monitoring Database and who is using it?

Notes:

CHAPTER #2: WHAT:

INTENT: What do I need to know about Terbinafine (OTC) (What will it do for me and what can I expect.)

1. What is the name of my Terbinafine (OTC) medication?

Notes:

2. What's the difference between all of the Terbinafine (OTC)'s class medications?

Notes:

3. What is the brand name for the drug Terbinafine (OTC)?

Notes:

4. What should you, as my doctor, know before prescribing Terbinafine (OTC) medication?

Notes:

5. What if Terbinafine (OTC) medication has changed since the application form was sent in?

Notes:

6. What is the evidence for this treatment?

Notes:

7. What about taking a new Terbinafine (OTC) medication?

Notes:

8. What to eat, or what to use as a medication together with Terbinafine (OTC)?

Notes:

9. What can parents and other adults do to help prevent prescription drug abuse among youth?

Notes:

10. What are the different treatment options?

Notes:

11. What is the way to get my life back on track, without the unwanted side effects of Terbinafine (OTC) prescription drugs?

Notes:

12. What if I'm already on medication and have side-effects from the Terbinafine (OTC)?

Notes:

13. What happens if I stop using Terbinafine (OTC) cold-turkey?

Notes:

14. What is the effect of Terbinafine (OTC) on

drowsiness?

Notes:

15. What are the side effects?

Notes:

16. What are the important warnings for males taking Terbinafine (OTC)?

Notes:

17. What questions haven't I asked that I should have?

Notes:

18. What Terbinafine (OTC) prescription drugs have serious side effects?

Notes:

19. What kind of medication will I have to take, Terbinafine (OTC) or anything else?

Notes:

20. What's to lose by trying another Terbinafine (OTC) class medication?

Notes:

21. What medications are available to treat my condition?

Notes:

22. What Terbinafine (OTC)'s class medication can I take best?

Notes:

23. What if my prescription Terbinafine (OTC) medication is lost or stolen?

Notes:

24. What about Terbinafine (OTC) prescription drug coverage?

Notes:

25. What are my options in relation to Terbinafine (OTC) medication, surgical procedures or remedy?

Notes:

26. At what point would you recommend Terbinafine (OTC) prescription drugs, alternative therapies, or surgery?

Notes:

27. What should I know about Terbinafine (OTC) medication?

Notes:

28. What about my current medications or allergies and the effect on it of Terbinafine (OTC)?

Notes:

29. What happens with my prescriptions for Terbinafine (OTC) medications while I am travelling overseas, how to get and fulfil those?

Notes:

30. What's your go-to question for your own doctor?

Notes:

31. What really works as well as these Terbinafine (OTC) medications, are there alternatives?

Notes:

32. What if I have tried various home remedies, over-the-counter medications or even Terbinafine (OTC) prescription medications with no help?

Notes:

33. What will this test tell us?

Notes:

34. What about Terbinafine (OTC)'s interactions with my medications?

Notes:

35. What will happen to me without Terbinafine (OTC) prescription drugs, diet, exercise, or nutritional supplements?

Notes:

36. What about side effects of Terbinafine (OTC)?

Notes:

37. What else could I be doing to stay healthy and prevent disease?

Notes:

38. Besides Terbinafine (OTC) medication, what else to do?

Notes:

39. What replacement medications can you suggest for Terbinafine (OTC)?

Notes:

40. What happens if I have to cut my Terbinafine (OTC) pills in half to make them last longer or skip a day of medication because I can't afford to buy it as often as it's prescribed?

Notes:

41. What should I do if I experience side effects from the Terbinafine (OTC)?

Notes:

42. What does this sign on my Terbinafine (OTC) prescription drug imply?

Notes:

43. What other prescription drugs should I avoid while taking my Terbinafine (OTC) medicines?

Notes:

44. What Terbinafine (OTC) medications are used?

Notes:

45. What medications can Terbinafine (OTC) interact with?

Notes:

46. What can I do to remember to take my Terbinafine (OTC) medication?

Notes:

47. What should I do if I miss my regular dose of Terbinafine (OTC)?

Notes:

48. What if I am unhappy with the results of Terbinafine (OTC) medication?

Notes:

49. What do you recommend to do with Terbinafine (OTC) medication adherence being difficult for me since my busy life pulls me in multiple directions - can you help me understand the ramifications of non-adherence?

Notes:

50. What types of Terbinafine (OTC) medications are available?

Notes:

51. What is my outcome?

Notes:

52. How will I benefit from working out in relation to my use of Terbinafine (OTC) prescription medication, and what type of exercise would you recommend?

Notes:

53. What are my options if I have difficulty paying for Terbinafine (OTC) prescription drugs?

Notes:

54. What about alcohol and its effect on Terbinafine (OTC) prescription drugs?

Notes:

55. Apart from Terbinafine (OTC) medication, what are other components of your management plan?

Notes:

56. What outcome should I expect?

Notes:

57. What if the Terbinafine (OTC) medications produce unwelcome or harmful effects?

Notes:

58. What medications should I ask for?

Notes:

59. What is a prescription drug error and how often and why do these errors occur??

Notes:

60. What would happen if I don't take the Terbinafine (OTC), would my health get worse?

Notes:

61. What will a positive result mean?

Notes:

62. What is a generic Terbinafine (OTC) medication or drug, what does that term mean and what can it do for me?

Notes:

63. Is it possible that my employer may look at what Terbinafine (OTC) prescription medications I'm taking?

Notes:

64. What is the nature of the Terbinafine (OTC) medications prescribed?

Notes:

65. What kind of Terbinafine (OTC) medications do the

varying plans offer and how much can I save?

Notes:

66. What's the probability that my Terbinafine (OTC) medication is causing my symptoms?

Notes:

67. What causes my condition?

Notes:

68. What is the safest way to dispose of unwanted medications?

Notes:

69. What are the side effects of the Terbinafine (OTC) medication?

Notes:

70. What kind of expectations should I have?

Notes:

71. In what way can mindfulness or meditation be useful?

Notes:

72. What is the best approach if I forget to take this Terbinafine (OTC) medication?

Notes:

73. What are the adverse health effects from Terbinafine (OTC) prescription drugs?

Notes:

74. What are the causes of Terbinafine (OTC) prescription drug abuse?

Notes:

75. What can I expect from Terbinafine (OTC) medication?

Notes:

76. What medications on the market, OTC or Terbinafine (OTC) prescription, can become harmful over time and would be dangerous if used well past the expiration date?

Notes:

77. What are some of the best non prescription medications I can give a try?

Notes:

78. What about my regular medications, any interference with Terbinafine (OTC)?

Notes:

79. What happens if I don't do anything?

Notes:

80. What are the signs and symptoms related to Terbinafine (OTC) addiction?

Notes:

81. What side effects can Terbinafine (OTC) medication cause?

Notes:

82. Can you help me understand how much of my Terbinafine (OTC) prescription drugs, equipment and services will be covered by my insurance and what I will have to pay?

Notes:

83. What if I'm taking other medication?

Notes:

84. What are the important warnings for females taking Terbinafine (OTC)?

Notes:

85. What if I have been taking Terbinafine (OTC) medication with little to no relief?

Notes:

86. What will be the net effect of Terbinafine (OTC) medications for me?

Notes:

87. What Terbinafine (OTC) medication should I take?

Notes:

88. What should I expect after a procedure in terms of soreness, what to watch for, Terbinafine (OTC) medication, bathing, and level of activity?

Notes:

89. What could be a natural alternative to more over-the-counter and Terbinafine (OTC) prescription drugs?

Notes:

90. What if Terbinafine (OTC) medication makes me gain weight?

Notes:

91. Is treatment required, if so - what is it?

Notes:

92. How do scientists determine whether the chemical compounds in Terbinafine (OTC) prescription medications do what they're claimed to do?

Notes:

93. What should I do if I have other prescription drug coverage and want to join Medicare First?

Notes:

94. What are the dosages of the Terbinafine (OTC) medication?

Notes:

95. Do I need to change what I eat or stop any Terbinafine (OTC) medications before doing a test?

Notes:

96. What will happen if I don't have the treatment?

Notes:

97. What other sources are available, who can I talk to about this?

Notes:

98. What can I do to help win the war on prescription drug abuse?

Notes:

99. What is the effect of Terbinafine (OTC) on infertility?

Notes:

100. How will you know what medications I am on?

Notes:

101. What sexual response side effects can I expect from these Terbinafine (OTC) medications?

Notes:

102. What if I am taking vitamins or over-the-counter drugs that could affect my Terbinafine (OTC) prescription drugs?

Notes:

103. I want to read more about my condition. What online sources should I trust?

Notes:

104. What are the Terbinafine (OTC) medications I can take?

Notes:

105. What is a 25/50 percent Terbinafine (OTC) prescription drug plan?

Notes:

106. What other drugs could interact with Terbinafine (OTC) medication?

Notes:

107. What are the benefits of having the test?

Notes:

108. What is my Terbinafine (OTC) prescription drug benefit?

Notes:

109. What sort of Terbinafine (OTC) prescription drug benefit is included?

Notes:

110. What are other treatment options?

Notes:

111. For what reasons would I have to be off Terbinafine (OTC) medication and for how long?

Notes:

112. Will I need medication and what will it be, Terbinafine (OTC) and/or anything else?

Notes:

113. What is the prescription drug of choice for breakthrough pain meds?

Notes:

114. What exactly leads one to get dependent on Terbinafine (OTC) prescription drugs?

Notes:

115. What lifestyle changes can change my condition?

Notes:

116. What types of vitamins and supplements should I be taking?

Notes:

117. How do I book in to have the test and what is the usual waiting period?

Notes:

118. What Terbinafine (OTC)-like medications are safe to take during pregnancy?

Notes:

119. What else can I do to treat my condition?

Notes:

120. What is the proper course of treatment for me?

Notes:

121. What prescription medications or off the shelf medicinal products would cause ringing in the ears?

Notes:

122. What's next?

Notes:

123. What if I take Terbinafine (OTC) prescription drugs and get little or no relief?

Notes:

124. What kind of experience with these issues do you have?

Notes:

125. What do I need to know about making the most of this Terbinafine (OTC) prescription?

Notes:

126. In what situation would I need to go for counseling if I'm receiving medication treatment?

Notes:

127. What is the branded prescription drug fee?

Notes:

128. What are your experiences with Terbinafine (OTC) prescription drugs?

Notes:

129. What prescription drugs are you yourself taking?

Notes:

130. What other Terbinafine (OTC)-like medications are in this class?

Notes:

131. What will my Terbinafine (OTC) medication do for me?

Notes:

132. What's the best mix for me of home remedies, over the counter (OTC) drugs and ointments and Terbinafine (OTC) prescription drugs?

Notes:

133. What is are food or drinks you recommend not to be taken with Terbinafine (OTC) prescription medications?

Notes:

134. What medications have you yourself used in the past to make yourself better?

Notes:

135. What are good reasons to not take my Terbinafine (OTC) prescription medication?

Notes:

136. What are my risks of accidentally taking an overdose of Terbinafine (OTC) prescription drugs?

Notes:

137. What are my Terbinafine (OTC) medication options?

Notes:

138. What non-Terbinafine (OTC) medications or vitamins should I take to speed up my healing?

Notes:

139. What does a Terbinafine (OTC) medication error involve?

Notes:

140. What are the Terbinafine (OTC) medication side-effects?

Notes:

141. What sources can I trust?

Notes:

142. What is Terbinafine (OTC) prescription drug detox?

Notes:

143. What kind of resources do I have available to me?

Notes:

144. What is the name of my condition, are there any other names it's known by?

Notes:

145. What if I have an allergic reaction to Terbinafine (OTC)?

Notes:

146. What if I am currently taking some other prescription medications?

Notes:

147. What is the safest way to dispose of unused prescription Terbinafine (OTC) medication?

Notes:

148. Is Terbinafine (OTC) safe when breastfeeding, what are the effects on nursing?

Notes:

149. What is a generic Terbinafine (OTC) medication?

Notes:

150. What will a negative result mean?

Notes:

151. What are your thoughts on hypnotherapy and Terbinafine (OTC)?

Notes:

152. What is the test for?

Notes:

153. What is the easiest way to obtain the latest information about Terbinafine (OTC) prescription drugs?

Notes:

154. What can I do to prevent my condition from recurring or worsening?

Notes:

155. What does my Terbinafine (OTC) medication look like?

Notes:

156. What is Terbinafine (OTC) medication for?

Notes:

157. What would you do if you were me?

Notes:

CHAPTER #3: WHERE:

INTENT: Where to next (Where can I find more information. Do i need a second opionion. What happens with tests.)

1. Does it matter at what time I use my Terbinafine (OTC) medication?

Notes:

2. Is there an effective herbal alternative or supplement to Terbinafine (OTC) medication?

Notes:

3. Which one of Terbinafine (OTC) medications is better for me than the others?

Notes:

4. Where can I find info about taking more than one prescription medications together with Terbinafine (OTC)?

Notes:

5. Do you have my vital records and medications up to date?

Notes:

6. Are all Terbinafine (OTC) prescription drugs covered under health care plans?

Notes:

7. Am I up to date on my routine health maintenance?

Notes:

8. What should I consider when buying coverage that provides prescription drug benefits?

Notes:

9. How do I safely discard Terbinafine (OTC) prescription drugs without having to worry?

Notes:

10. Is there a possibility of reaction to Terbinafine (OTC) medications?

Notes:

11. Will taking Terbinafine (OTC) make me irritable?

Notes:

12. Is this necessary right now?

Notes:

13. What exactly is this Terbinafine (OTC) medication for in my case and how do you think it is working so well?

Notes:

14. Should I take my Terbinafine (OTC) medications at a regular time each day?

Notes:

15. Are the supplements I take worthwhile?

Notes:

16. Is Terbinafine (OTC) medication a substitute for therapy?

Notes:

17. How do I avoid getting in a place where I need so many prescription drugs to function?

Notes:

18. What if my current Terbinafine (OTC) prescription drugs are not on the formulary or are limited on the formulary?

Notes:

19. Where would I store my Terbinafine (OTC)

medications?

Notes:

20. Will Terbinafine (OTC) cause a mood change?

Notes:

21. Who monitors the safety and effectiveness of Terbinafine (OTC) prescription drugs?

Notes:

22. If I have been taking the same prescription drugs for a long time, when is it time to evaluate?

Notes:

23. How do Terbinafine (OTC) prescription drugs work?

Notes:

24. Should I bring a copy of my prescription medications?

Notes:

25. Do younger people need less of the Terbinafine (OTC) medication than older people?

Notes:

26. What if I am out of the country and lose my Terbinafine (OTC) prescription medications?

Notes:

27. Will Terbinafine (OTC) medication control my symptoms adequately?

Notes:

28. Terbinafine (OTC) is most definitely a prescription drug?

Notes:

29. Where would you send your partner or children?

Notes:

30. Is Terbinafine (OTC) medication the only answer for me?

Notes:

31. Where are others buying their Terbinafine (OTC) prescription medications?

Notes:

32. What do you turn to for adjunctive medications, usually?

Notes:

33. Do Terbinafine (OTC) medications deliver on their promise?

Notes:

34. Can I take Terbinafine (OTC) with my current medications?

Notes:

35. Will Terbinafine (OTC) interfere with other prescription medications?

Notes:

36. Because Medicare prescription drug coverage is so new to me, where can I get aid deciding on a program?

Notes:

37. How to take Terbinafine (OTC) medication?

Notes:

38. Which Terbinafine (OTC)-like medication gives the most rapid relief?

Notes:

39. What is a 3-Tier or 4-Tier prescription drug plan?

Notes:

40. Will these Terbinafine (OTC) medications cause weight gain?

Notes:

41. If remedies help, what is the nature of Terbinafine (OTC) medications and where could one go to explore them?

Notes:

42. Is Terbinafine (OTC) as effective as other prescription medications?

Notes:

43. Where are Terbinafine (OTC) prescription drug users getting their prescription filled locally?

Notes:

44. Can you suggest alternatives to Terbinafine (OTC) prescription medication?

Notes:

45. Should I rely on Terbinafine (OTC), natural cures or over the counter medication?

Notes:

46. What do each of these Terbinafine (OTC) prescription medications have in common?

Notes:

47. Is it all right for me to take allergy medication?

Notes:

48. How do I use my insurance to get discounts on my Terbinafine (OTC) prescription medication?

Notes:

49. Do Terbinafine (OTC) medications accelerate aging?

Notes:

50. Are there other remedies, is there any relief other

than Terbinafine (OTC) Medication?

Notes:

51. Will any of the supplements that have been prescribed for me interfere with any Terbinafine (OTC) prescription medications I may already be on?

Notes:

52. Are non-prescription drugs less effective than Terbinafine (OTC)?

Notes:

53. What should I do if my symptoms are not relieved while taking Terbinafine (OTC) medication?

Notes:

54. Will Terbinafine (OTC) interact with any other medicines I take - including any vitamins - herbal medicine or other complementary medicine?

Notes:

55. Would increasing the dose of Terbinafine (OTC) have a positive effect or would I be better off asking you to try some new medications?

Notes:

56. Will any supplements interact with my Terbinafine (OTC) prescription drugs?

Notes:

57. Are there any contraindications with Terbinafine (OTC) to other medications?

Notes:

58. Are my Terbinafine (OTC) medications safe to use while breastfeeding?

Notes:

59. Which prescription medications can cause impotence?

Notes:

60. Where should I get my Terbinafine (OTC) prescription drugs?

Notes:

61. Are Terbinafine (OTC) medications effective?

Notes:

62. Where can I get more info about that?

Notes:

63. Will Terbinafine (OTC) have an effect on nausea?

Notes:

64. If I use prescription drugs, can I be arrested for DUI?

Notes:

65. Where do I go if I've run out of money and desperately need Terbinafine (OTC) medication or a medical procedure?

Notes:

66. Can I continue to take Terbinafine (OTC) prescription drugs over 10, 20 and 30 years or more?

Notes:

67. Do I have to be on more medications because of the side effects of Terbinafine (OTC)?

Notes:

68. Can assisted living patients receive 90-day supplies of medications?

Notes:

69. Are any nutrients depleted by this Terbinafine (OTC) medication?

Notes:

70. Is it possible to lower my blood pressure without taking prescription drugs?

Notes:

71. Are there medications available that really fix the underlying cause of my condition?

Notes:

72. Will you try and keep my Terbinafine (OTC) medications at a level where I can function?

Notes:

73. Do I need this particular Terbinafine (OTC) medication?

Notes:

74. Have you instructed patients to discontinue taking their Terbinafine (OTC), or other prescription drugs?

Notes:

75. Are there any other precautions or warnings for this Terbinafine (OTC) medication?

Notes:

76. Can I take over-the-counter drugs or are prescription drugs more effective?

Notes:

77. Where can I get my Terbinafine (OTC) prescription medications filled?

Notes:

78. Should I be worried about this lump/spot/____?

Notes:

79. Can I use this app I found?

Notes:

80. What is this Terbinafine (OTC) medication for, why am I taking it?

Notes:

81. Please explain, what are the differences between

generic and brand Terbinafine (OTC) medications?

Notes:

82. Does my plan have a Terbinafine (OTC) prescription drug formulary?

Notes:

83. If I need a surgery and I did go ahead with the surgery, how might that affect the Terbinafine (OTC) medications I take?

Notes:

CHAPTER #4: WHEN:

INTENT: When should I take or stop taking Terbinafine (OTC) and how (When should I take it, stop taking it and how.)

1. Is it possible to start with a solution which is natural and effective and less expensive than Terbinafine (OTC) prescription medication?

Notes:

2. Are generics available for all Terbinafine (OTC) prescription drugs?

Notes:

3. Can Reiki be used when taking Terbinafine (OTC) medications?

Notes:

4. I take daily prescription medications, may I take my pills before I have my blood drawn?

Notes:

5. When does Terbinafine (OTC) medication begin working?

Notes:

6. When is it appropriate and safe to prescribe Terbinafine (OTC) medication for my condition?

Notes:

7. When does this Terbinafine (OTC) medication expire?

Notes:

8. Can Canadian drug pharmacies mail my Terbinafine (OTC) prescription drugs and medications to me?

Notes:

9. Do you have research you can share on Terbinafine (OTC) prescription drug prices?

Notes:

10. Is my weight okay?

Notes:

11. Do pill boxes help prevent Terbinafine (OTC) medication errors?

Notes:

12. Should I review my Medicare prescription drug plan choice every year?

Notes:

13. If there is an all new Terbinafine (OTC) medication that comes up how can it have been adequately tested in terms of it's long term negative effects?

Notes:

14. Are there generic equivalents available for my Terbinafine (OTC) prescription drugs?

Notes:

15. When you prescribe Terbinafine (OTC) prescription medication for my condition, how do you weigh the side effects?

Notes:

16. Are these Terbinafine (OTC) medications really helping?

Notes:

17. Where does my Terbinafine (OTC) prescription medication come from?

Notes:

18. Does my policy cover Terbinafine (OTC) prescription drugs?

Notes:

19. If I am taking Terbinafine (OTC) prescription medications can I take natural remedies?

Notes:

20. Should I get a second opinion?

Notes:

21. Is Terbinafine (OTC) compatible with my current prescribed medication?

Notes:

22. When should I stop using Terbinafine (OTC) medication because of....?

Notes:

23. When I have been on the same amount of Terbinafine (OTC) medication for years – when should that be re-evaluated?

Notes:

24. What are some great ways to help remind me when to take Terbinafine (OTC) medications?

Notes:

25. Will I be able to do _____ after treatment?

Notes:

26. Do I HAVE to be on Terbinafine (OTC) medication?

Notes:

27. How do I deal with any Terbinafine (OTC) prescription medication when a side effect may be stated as 'may cause nausea or vomiting'?

Notes:

28. Are there any known Terbinafine (OTC) prescription medication and chia seeds side effects when they are combined?

Notes:

29. How does a Terbinafine (OTC) medication reminder service work?

Notes:

30. What does one do when the only real help, the only Terbinafine (OTC) medication available, no longer works?

Notes:

31. Can my condition come back?

Notes:

32. Is it safe getting pregnant while on Terbinafine (OTC) medications?

Notes:

33. Is it okay to take my Terbinafine (OTC) prescription drugs and multivitamin during a fast?

Notes:

34. Will my gender or ethnic group be denied

Terbinafine (OTC) medications that work better for other groups but not for my ethnic or gender group?

Notes:

35. What is the effect of my Terbinafine (OTC) use if I smoke?

Notes:

36. Should I be worried about getting the wrong interaction if I combine Terbinafine (OTC) prescription drugs with natural supplements?

Notes:

37. Will my Terbinafine (OTC) prescription drugs build up toxins in my body?

Notes:

38. Is it safe and legal to buy Terbinafine (OTC) prescription drugs and other medications abroad?

Notes:

39. What medications do I need to stop and when?

Notes:

40. Can I travel to _____ with prescription drugs used as medication for my condition?

Notes:

41. When should I take this Terbinafine (OTC) medicine?

Notes:

42. Can I take Terbinafine (OTC) with my other medications?

Notes:

43. Should I be on Terbinafine (OTC) medication?

Notes:

44. Can I drink alcohol while I am taking Terbinafine (OTC)?

Notes:

45. When did you graduate from medical school?

Notes:

46. What would happen if I were suddenly unable to get access to my Terbinafine (OTC) prescription drugs?

Notes:

47. How/when do I get test results?

Notes:

48. Can nutritional yeasts, especially brewers yeast, interact with Terbinafine (OTC) medications?

Notes:

49. Can my child have his or her Terbinafine (OTC) medication administered during the school day?

Notes:

50. Can I take the generic version of your prescription drugs?

Notes:

51. If I get sick - will you see me in the hospital?

Notes:

52. Can enzymes be taken with other Terbinafine (OTC) prescription medications?

Notes:

53. What f I have any allergies to food, medications or things in the environment?

Notes:

54. How and when should I take my Terbinafine (OTC) medication?

Notes:

55. Are there health insurers who reimburse for

Terbinafine (OTC) prescription drugs based on how well they work?

Notes:

56. Are there simpler - safer options?

Notes:

57. Should I stop taking that Terbinafine (OTC) medication?

Notes:

58. Can I safely use natural remedies and Terbinafine (OTC) prescription drugs together?

Notes:

59. Can I take Terbinafine (OTC) medication?

Notes:

60. When should I stop taking Terbinafine (OTC) medication?

Notes:

61. Are any medications I am taking dangerous for my stage of this disease?

Notes:

62. If I take Terbinafine (OTC) prescription drugs long term, do I run the risk of becoming addicted?

Notes:

63. When will I know that I am taking excessive pain medication?

Notes:

64. Do you know of any medications available out there that would help me be more comfortable?

Notes:

65. Will you try and reach the primary reason for my problem before prescribing Terbinafine (OTC) medications to solve my particular signs and symptoms?

Notes:

66. Um - can you explain that again?

Notes:

67. Do Terbinafine (OTC) prescription drugs create new mental problems?

Notes:

68. When can seniors join a Terbinafine (OTC) prescription drug plan?

Notes:

69. Will Terbinafine (OTC) prescription medications cause weight loss?

Notes:

70. Is sharing Terbinafine (OTC) prescription drugs illegal?

Notes:

71. Is it either / or when it comes to natural medicines and Terbinafine (OTC) prescription drugs?

Notes:

72. Can you help me save money on my Terbinafine (OTC) prescription medication?

Notes:

73. If you have a Terbinafine (OTC) prescription drug in your pocket, outside of the container when arrested is that considered DUI?

Notes:

74. When could Terbinafine (OTC) medication not be working anymore?

Notes:

75. What does 50 deductible for brand name prescription drugs mean?

Notes:

76. When might herbal and nutritional therapies be a good alternative to over-the-counter and Terbinafine (OTC) prescription medications for people with my condition?

Notes:

77. Is this necessary now?

Notes:

78. If I do therapy, can I change or stop my Terbinafine (OTC) medications?

Notes:

79. Is there a better way to easily adhere to Terbinafine (OTC) prescription medication regimens?

Notes:

80. Will I require any Terbinafine (OTC) prescription drugs?

Notes:

81. Where can I obtain a list of Terbinafine (OTC) prescription drugs that require prior approval?

Notes:

82. When and how will I get the results?

Notes:

83. When should I be on Terbinafine (OTC) medication?

Notes:

CHAPTER #5: WHY:

INTENT: Why do I need Terbinafine (OTC)
(Are there Alternatives. Why do I need
it. Which symptoms does it medicate.)

1. Why are you giving me a blood test - and what will the results tell us?

Notes:

2. What if I am currently without prescription drug coverage?

Notes:

3. Why can't I buy some prescription drugs online?

Notes:

4. How long am I expected to take this Terbinafine (OTC) medication?

Notes:

5. Why would I need Terbinafine (OTC) prescription medication reminders?

Notes:

6. Where can I buy Terbinafine (OTC) prescription drugs cheaper?

Notes:

7. Why and when use acupuncture for treating pain instead of, or combined with, taking pain medication?

Notes:

8. Is self-administration of Terbinafine (OTC) medication allowed?

Notes:

9. How can you help me when I suffer from chronic pain, but am leery about taking prescription medication to help it?

Notes:

10. Do we have to do this test now?

Notes:

11. How long will I need to take this Terbinafine (OTC) medication?

Notes:

12. Are there any drug interactions if Terbinafine (OTC) is taken in combination with other medications?

Notes:

13. Why do I need to manage Terbinafine (OTC) medications?

Notes:

14. Where else can I go for Terbinafine (OTC) prescription medication, what are my options?

Notes:

15. **Can I schedule my surgery for the morning?**

Notes:

16. **Should I bring a list of medications and allergies?**

Notes:

17. Should I be concerned about all the Terbinafine (OTC) medication I need to take to stay on top of my health problems?

Notes:

18. Why do I need Terbinafine (OTC) medicine?

Notes:

19. Will I be on Terbinafine (OTC) medication forever?

Notes:

20. Why is it important to take my Terbinafine (OTC) prescription medication exactly as prescribed?

Notes:

21. Are there any counter-indications about taking this supplement while taking any prescription drugs?

Notes:

22. Will I be able to carry enough prescription medications to avoid any health emergencies?

Notes:

23. Can Terbinafine (OTC) cause me to get a dry mouth as side effect?

Notes:

24. Is it necessary to refill my Terbinafine (OTC) medication repeatedly annually?

Notes:

25. Are there any other restrictions on Terbinafine (OTC) prescription drug coverage?

Notes:

26. Why is buying Terbinafine (OTC) prescription drugs without a prescription dangerous?

Notes:

27. Can I take Terbinafine (OTC) with other medications?

Notes:

28. Will taking Terbinafine (OTC) medication effect my mission call?

Notes:

29. How will the treatment effect the medications that I currently take for _____?

Notes:

30. Should I take Terbinafine (OTC) with food or drink?

Notes:

31. Why does a prescription drug require authorization by a qualified professional and others do not?

Notes:

32. Can I ever be free of having to use prescription drugs?

Notes:

33. Will St. John's Wort interfere with Terbinafine (OTC) prescription medications?

Notes:

34. Is Terbinafine (OTC) a slow releasing medication?

Notes:

35. Do you offer treatment programs for those suffering from Terbinafine (OTC) prescription drug addiction?

Notes:

36. Is this something I should worry about or is it just a side effect of Terbinafine (OTC)?

Notes:

37. What are the best ways that do not require prescription medications to fall asleep faster?

Notes:

38. Why is Terbinafine (OTC) medication prescribed?

Notes:

39. Should I stop my Terbinafine (OTC) medications before any procedure?

Notes:

40. Why are Terbinafine (OTC) medications so popular?

Notes:

41. When is it time to think about why I'm on these Terbinafine (OTC) drugs?

Notes:

42. Is switching from one biologic medication to another effective?

Notes:

43. What is the difference between brand name medication and their generic counter parts?

Notes:

44. Why are we doing these tests?

Notes:

45. Are there other Terbinafine (OTC)-like medications to relieve this discomfort?

Notes:

46. Are all drug-drug interactions limited to Terbinafine (OTC) prescription medications?

Notes:

47. What treatments, therapies and medications are recommended or available for my condition?

Notes:

48. Is there an alternative medication?

Notes:

49. Are there any supplements or Terbinafine (OTC) medications?

Notes:

50. Why is Terbinafine (OTC) a prescription drug?

Notes:

51. Why is this Terbinafine (OTC) medication prescribed?

Notes:

52. Is Terbinafine (OTC) a medicine with real evidence?

Notes:

53. Can the Terbinafine (OTC) medication cause substance abuse?

Notes:

54. Do I take Terbinafine (OTC) prescription medications every day?

Notes:

55. Are there any side effects associated with this Terbinafine (OTC) medication that I should know about?

Notes:

56. What happens if I am willing to try new medications if the current Terbinafine (OTC) ones are not working?

Notes:

57. Is it legal to buy Terbinafine (OTC) prescription medications online?

Notes:

58. Why would I, while regularly taking prescription medications, have to approach grapefruit consumption with caution?

Notes:

59. Can you take expired Terbinafine (OTC) medications or not?

Notes:

60. Will any tests be necessary while I am taking Terbinafine (OTC) medication?

Notes:

61. Can Terbinafine (OTC) be mixed with other medications, dietary supplements, or alcohol?

Notes:

62. Why does my family's medical history matter, and what should I do about it?

Notes:

63. Will my body get to depend upon a certain amount of my Terbinafine (OTC) prescription drug, an amount that grows higher the longer I am on the drug?

Notes:

64. Why have my bowel habits/appetite/mood/sex drive/etc changed?

Notes:

65. Can I take _____ with Terbinafine (OTC) prescription drugs?

Notes:

66. Can you help me with finding the money to purchase doctor visits and also Terbinafine (OTC) prescriptions medication?

Notes:

67. Will my Terbinafine (OTC) prescription drug have a drivers warning on it?

Notes:

68. Do enzymes interfere with Terbinafine (OTC) prescription drugs?

Notes:

69. Do I need a change in my Terbinafine (OTC) medication?

Notes:

70. How will I know when my Terbinafine (OTC) medications are working?

Notes:

71. Can Terbinafine (OTC) medications or my health problems keep me awake?

Notes:

72. Can people be guilty of DUI if they are driving under the influence of Terbinafine (OTC) prescription medications?

Notes:

73. How do I get my Terbinafine (OTC) medication without prescription drug coverage?

Notes:

74. Is there a generic version of the Terbinafine (OTC) medication?

Notes:

75. If I take a Terbinafine (OTC) medication, will it require more medication to counter the side effects?

Notes:

76. Where can I make cost savings?

Notes:

**77. Is it probable to uncover how to deal with
_____ without taking prescription medication?**

Notes:

78. Could you write it down?

Notes:

79. Are Terbinafine (OTC) prescription medications
included in my monthly insurance fee?

Notes:

80. Can or should I take my Terbinafine (OTC)
medications at breakfast with my grapefruit juice?

Notes:

81. Why go the Terbinafine (OTC) medication route?

Notes:

82. Could I have afforded it without Terbinafine (OTC) prescription drug insurance?

Notes:

83. Why are you doing this test?

Notes:

CHAPTER #6: HOW:

INTENT: How will Terbinafine (OTC) affect me (How will it affect me negatively. How do I know if its a problem for me.)

1. How do I dispose of Terbinafine (OTC) prescription medications?

Notes:

2. How often will I take the Terbinafine (OTC) medication?

Notes:

3. How does Terbinafine (OTC) interact with other medications?

Notes:

4. So how do I save money on my Terbinafine (OTC) prescription drugs?

Notes:

5. State prescription drug price web sites, how useful are they to me as a Terbinafine (OTC) consumer?

Notes:

6. How are Terbinafine (OTC) prescription drugs abused?

Notes:

7. How long does the Terbinafine (OTC) medication last?

Notes:

8. How long will I need the treatment for?

Notes:

9. How can I make sure I am sufficiently stocked with the Terbinafine (OTC) prescription medications I need?

Notes:

10. How can I support my bone health naturally with and without medication?

Notes:

11. How will Terbinafine (OTC) affect my sleeping pattern?

Notes:

12. How serious is this condition?

Notes:

13. How can I opt for the generic alternative Terbinafine (OTC) medication that gives me the exact same results?

Notes:

14. How many patients with my condition have you treated?

Notes:

15. How should I take this Terbinafine (OTC) medication?

Notes:

16. How about a new Terbinafine (OTC)-like prescription drug?

Notes:

17. How should I use this Terbinafine (OTC) medication?

Notes:

18. How do I know if I have permanent hair loss due to medication?

Notes:

19. How can I reduce or stop some of my

medications?

Notes:

20. How do I read the label on my Terbinafine (OTC) prescription drug package?

Notes:

21. How's my weight?

Notes:

22. How will Terbinafine (OTC) affect the other medications that I'm taking?

Notes:

23. How can I dispose of my Terbinafine (OTC) prescription drugs safely?

Notes:

24. How will I hear about my test results?

Notes:

25. How do I take this Terbinafine (OTC) medication?

Notes:

26. How do you handle children on Terbinafine (OTC) medication?

Notes:

27. How long does a Terbinafine (OTC) medication remain active in your body?

Notes:

28. How does a person with dementia, living alone, manage her Terbinafine (OTC) medication?

Notes:

29. How is Terbinafine (OTC) medication supposed to help me?

Notes:

30. How can I reduce my Terbinafine (OTC) prescription drug costs?

Notes:

31. How do different Terbinafine (OTC)-class prescription medications work differently?

Notes:

32. So I got a condition and a Terbinafine (OTC) medication – how am I, as a patient, supposed to manage treatment?

Notes:

33. How long do I have to take Terbinafine (OTC) medication?

Notes:

34. How long will it take to get the results?

Notes:

35. How long do I need to take the Terbinafine (OTC) medicine for?

Notes:

36. Are there support groups for people with this problem and how would I contact them?

Notes:

37. How soon should I come back?

Notes:

38. How many surgeries do you perform each year?

Notes:

39. How is the test done?

Notes:

40. How to store Terbinafine (OTC) medication?

Notes:

41. How common is Terbinafine (OTC) prescription drug abuse?

Notes:

42. My Terbinafine (OTC) medications, just how safe are they?

Notes:

43. How long does the prescription drug Terbinafine (OTC) stay in your system?

Notes:

44. How will I know if the Terbinafine (OTC) prescription and over-the-counter medications I take are interacting properly?

Notes:

45. Do you know how long it will take me to get my Terbinafine (OTC) medication?

Notes:

46. How do generic medications compare in quality to brand name drugs?

Notes:

47. How wide-ranging is the Terbinafine (OTC) prescription drug coverage?

Notes:

48. How quickly do I have to start the treatment?

Notes:

49. So how do you know if you, or someone you love is having problems with Terbinafine (OTC) prescription drug abuse?

Notes:

50. How do I get better without Terbinafine (OTC) medication?

Notes:

51. How soon do I need to have the test?

Notes:

52. How can Terbinafine (OTC) prescription drug abuse be recognized and stopped?

Notes:

53. How often do I need to have the test done?

Notes:

54. How long is it likely to last?

Notes:

55. Will Terbinafine (OTC) interact with my current medications?

Notes:

56. How should I take my Terbinafine (OTC) medication?

Notes:

57. How can Terbinafine (OTC) medication be detected?

Notes:

58. How do I manage my Terbinafine (OTC) medications?

Notes:

59. How effective is this treatment?

Notes:

60. How do I manage multiple prescription medications together with Terbinafine (OTC)?

Notes:

61. How does Terbinafine (OTC) prescription drug abuse start?

Notes:

62. Are there drugs to lift my mood, and how can this be achieved without prescription medications?

Notes:

63. How to go about it if I want to use a lower dosage of Terbinafine (OTC)?

Notes:

64. How do we order or pick up Terbinafine (OTC) medications?

Notes:

65. How should I dispose of Terbinafine (OTC) prescription drugs?

Notes:

66. How should this Terbinafine (OTC) medication be stored?

Notes:

67. How can I find a few methods that can help my condition without the use of Terbinafine (OTC) prescription medication?

Notes:

68. How long should I take Terbinafine (OTC) medication?

Notes:

69. How should this Terbinafine (OTC) medication be taken?

Notes:

70. How will I know if my current Terbinafine (OTC) Prescription Drug coverage is as good as the new Medicare Terbinafine (OTC) Prescription Drug coverage?

Notes:

71. Is there an Over-The-Counter Medication that helps or maybe even can replace my Terbinafine (OTC)

Prescription Medication?

Notes:

72. How will I feel when I'm on Terbinafine (OTC) medications?

Notes:

73. How can my mental state successfully improve using medication or therapy?

Notes:

74. Can I expect any side effects from my Terbinafine (OTC) medication?

Notes:

75. How will I get the test results?

Notes:

76. How long will the effect of Terbinafine (OTC) medication last?

Notes:

77. How is the Terbinafine (OTC) medication delivered?

Notes:

78. Is it probable to find out how to deal with my condition without taking Terbinafine (OTC) prescription drugs?

Notes:

79. How do the police suspect impairment by Terbinafine (OTC) prescription medication?

Notes:

80. How can I learn more about my symptoms or condition?

Notes:

81. In case I need pain relief, how can I get access to medical cannabis?

Notes:

82. How often is the Terbinafine (OTC) medication taken?

Notes:

83. How accurate are the results of the test?

Notes:

CHAPTER #7: HOW MUCH:

INTENT: How much will taking
Terbinafine (OTC) cost me (In money and
Terbinafine (OTC)'s effect on quality of
life.)

1. I feel like I need more medication, will you as my doctor be able to support me with my requests?

Notes:

2. Are you aware of my personal medical history including current medications, allergies, and other considerations or limitations?

Notes:

3. Should I join a Medicare Prescription Drug Plan even if I don't take many prescription drugs?

Notes:

4. Can alternative medicine counter Terbinafine (OTC) prescription medication and over-the-counters with their limited effectiveness and potential side effects?

Notes:

5. Can using too much or too little Terbinafine (OTC) prescription drugs harm my health?

Notes:

6. How much will the test cost?

Notes:

7. Are Terbinafine (OTC) medications safe for young kids?

Notes:

8. Will the cost be covered by Medicare - my concession or Veterans Affairs card or by private health insurance?

Notes:

9. Will I feel doped from Terbinafine (OTC)?

Notes:

10. Which Terbinafine (OTC)'s class related medication is the safest for me?

Notes:

11. Can the nurse see me?

Notes:

12. May an employer ask all employees what prescription medications they are taking?

Notes:

13. Does my plan cover my Terbinafine (OTC) prescription drugs?

Notes:

14. If acupuncture improves my condition, can I stop taking Terbinafine (OTC) prescription medications?

Notes:

15. Does switching Terbinafine (OTC) prescription drugs to over the counter as I age have any negative side effects?

Notes:

16. Is there a Medicare Advantage plan provider who will cover my Terbinafine (OTC) prescription drug costs during the donut hole?

Notes:

17. Is it normal to feel this way?

Notes:

18. How much experience with this test or procedure do you have?

Notes:

19. Can certain over the counter medications or Terbinafine (OTC) prescription medications cause a false positive for illegal drugs in a blood test?

Notes:

20. Do some Terbinafine (OTC) prescription drugs cost more or have additional requirements for coverage?

Notes:

21. Can I take this Terbinafine (OTC) medicine if I am pregnant?

Notes:

22. How to get my Terbinafine (OTC) medication increased?

Notes:

23. How do I get the Medicare Terbinafine (OTC) prescription drug benefit?

Notes:

24. How does my child at an out-of-state school obtain prescription drugs?

Notes:

25. What are the active ingredients in Terbinafine (OTC) prescription medication?

Notes:

26. How do prescription medications compare to herbal forms of treatment for my condition?

Notes:

27. Can we really know what is in Terbinafine (OTC) prescription drugs?

Notes:

28. How much am I likely to spend on Terbinafine (OTC) prescription drugs?

Notes:

29. Can Terbinafine (OTC) prescription drugs cause problems during pregnancy?

Notes:

30. What should you do if I've messed up with my Terbinafine (OTC) medication?

Notes:

31. How much Terbinafine (OTC) prescription medication can I order from my pharmacy at one time?

Notes:

32. Are nutritional supplements safe to take if I am taking Terbinafine (OTC) prescription medications?

Notes:

33. Do you think that I may have or get a problem with Terbinafine (OTC) medications?

Notes:

34. Is there a non-prescription Terbinafine (OTC) medication you might recommend?

Notes:

35. How much will my Terbinafine (OTC) prescription drugs cost me?

Notes:

36. Can you inform me about nutrition, exercise, Terbinafine (OTC) medications and complications?

Notes:

37. How much do the Terbinafine (OTC) prescription drugs cost in this plan as compared to other plans?

Notes:

38. What does using a prescription drug Off-label mean?

Notes:

39. How does herb _____ compare to, or has an

effect on, Terbinafine (OTC) prescription drugs?

Notes:

40. How much will this cost me?

Notes:

41. So, is this a 'wow-factor' Terbinafine (OTC) medication?

Notes:

42. Should I take medication to lower my blood pressure?

Notes:

43. Is there a certain Terbinafine (OTC) or other medication that can improve my symptoms?

Notes:

44. Should I really use this Terbinafine (OTC) medication?

Notes:

45. How much will the plan cover for Terbinafine (OTC) prescription drugs?

Notes:

46. Could natural products be just as effective as Terbinafine (OTC) prescription medications?

Notes:

47. Can I take _____ with Terbinafine (OTC) prescription drugs?

Notes:

48. How much does Terbinafine (OTC) cost?

Notes:

49. Should I lock up my Terbinafine (OTC) prescription drugs?

Notes:

50. Where can US citizens buy their prescription drugs online from legally, in confidence, and under which conditions?

Notes:

51. How much Terbinafine (OTC) medication can be brought through customs in case I travel?

Notes:

52. Will Medicare be enough to cover the cost of my medical care, especially Terbinafine (OTC) prescription drugs?

Notes:

53. Is it covered by Medicare - my concession or Veterans Affairs card or my private health insurance?

Notes:

54. Can you explain my options for Medicare, Medicare/Medicaid, Disability, Supplemental Insurance, Part D Prescription Drug Plans, or

Medicare Billings?

Notes:

55. How much will it cost, will the cost be covered by the PBS - my concession or Veterans Affairs card or by private health insurance?

Notes:

56. Am I am worrying too much?

Notes:

57. How much will the treatment cost?

Notes:

58. Can Terbinafine (OTC) medication cause hair loss?

Notes:

59. Are there any risks or side effects?

Notes:

60. How much should I be charged for my Terbinafine (OTC) prescription medications?

Notes:

61. Is Terbinafine (OTC) safe if taking medications for high blood pressure?

Notes:

62. Could any of the Terbinafine (OTC) medications contribute to impotence?

Notes:

63. How do I know how much my Terbinafine (OTC) prescription medication will be?

Notes:

64. Does Terbinafine (OTC) medication work?

Notes:

65. How much can I use this Terbinafine (OTC) prescription drug plan?

Notes:

66. Which Terbinafine (OTC) medications are addictive?

Notes:

67. Do I need to prepare for the test (for example - by fasting beforehand)?

Notes:

68. How much do I need to really understand about the interactions of my Terbinafine (OTC) prescription drugs?

Notes:

69. Will kinesiology interfere with Terbinafine (OTC) medication?

Notes:

70. Which part of Medicare will cover my Terbinafine (OTC) prescription drugs?

Notes:

71. Will it help when I tell you about all my current medications and vitamin and herbal supplements?

Notes:

72. Regarding dosage, exactly how much of Terbinafine (OTC) can I take?

Notes:

73. Precisely what are some good reasons Terbinafine (OTC) prescription drugs can be recommended?

Notes:

74. Are you considering a trial of Terbinafine (OTC) medications and/or anything else?

Notes:

75. Which method of Terbinafine (OTC) prescription

medication detox is best?

Notes:

76. Do Terbinafine (OTC) medications work for everybody?

Notes:

77. Just how much do you know about the numerous types of Terbinafine (OTC) medications for the different types of my condition?

Notes:

78. How much is Medicare Terbinafine (OTC) prescription drug coverage worth?

Notes:

79. How much does it normally cost to get the surgery done, including all Terbinafine (OTC) medications and tests (ultrasounds,x-rays,medicines, hospital stay)?

Notes:

80. What if I take pain medication for _____ ?

Notes:

81. Does the Terbinafine (OTC) medicine need to be stored in the fridge?

Notes:

82. Does Terbinafine (OTC) medication and therapy work together?

Notes:

83. Should I take Terbinafine (OTC) with other medications?

Notes:

Index

145

Please 70
pocket 86
police 121
policies 13
policy 75
popular 97
positive 21, 36, 66, 127
possible 36, 68, 72
potent 18
potential 18, 124
precaution 1
precise 1
Precisely 137
pregnancy 47, 129
pregnant 78, 127
prepare 4, 136
prepared 5
prescribe 1, 73, 75
prescribed 10, 32, 36, 65, 76, 93, 96, 99
prescribes 3
preserve 12
pressing 4
pressure 68, 131, 135
prevent 8, 26, 31, 54, 74
prices 16, 74
primary 84
private 124, 133-134
proactive 3
probable 104, 121
problem 5, 84, 106, 113, 129
problems 8, 85, 92, 103, 115, 129
procedure 41, 67, 96, 126
procedures 3, 29
process 3
produce 35
product 1, 3
products 1, 47, 132
program 62
programs 96
promise 61
proper 47
properly 114
provider 126

providers   3, 5
provides   5, 56
providing   3
publisher   1
purchase   3, 102
purchased   3
qualified   8, 95
quality 3, 115, 123
question   2-3, 6, 30
questions   3-5, 27
quickly 115
reaction   52, 57
really   16, 30, 69, 75, 128, 131, 136
reason 5, 84
reasons   45, 50, 137
receive   8, 17, 68
receiving   48
recently   3
recognized   116
recommend   19, 29, 33-34, 50, 130
recording   1
records   9, 56
recurring   54
reduce 109, 112
references   140
refill   93
refuse   10
regarding   1, 8, 137
regimen   10
regimens   87
regular 33, 39, 58
regularly   100
reimburse   82
related 18, 39, 125
-related   14
relation   29, 34
releasing   95
relevant   3
relief   40, 48, 62, 64, 121
relieve 97
relieved   65
religion 14
remain 111

system 114
taking 7-8, 11, 16, 19, 22, 25, 27, 32, 36, 40, 44, 46, 49-50, 52, 56-57, 59, 65, 68-70, 72, 76, 80, 83-84, 90-91, 93-94, 100, 104, 110, 121, 123, 125-126, 129, 135
Talking 3
tested 74
therapies   29, 87, 98
therapy   58, 87, 120, 139
things 4, 82
thought   19
thoughts   53
through   133
throughout   1
together   25, 56, 83, 117, 139
topical 18
toxins 79
trademark   1
trademarks   1
trained 1
travel 80, 133
travelling   29
treated   109
treating   90
treatment   10, 25-26, 42-43, 45, 47-48, 77, 94, 96, 107, 112, 115, 117, 128, 134
treatments   14, 98
trying 28
typically   8, 22
unable 10, 81
uncover   104
underlying   10, 69
understand   33, 40, 136
unhappy   33
unused 52
unwanted   26, 37
unwelcome   35
useful 38, 107
usually 61
validating   7
various 21, 30
varying 37
version 21, 82, 103, 140
Veterans   124, 133-134

Printed in Great Britain
by Amazon